Relieving Irritable Bowel Syndrome Naturally

Bishop Dr. Juliette D. Fagan

Naturopathic Practitioner

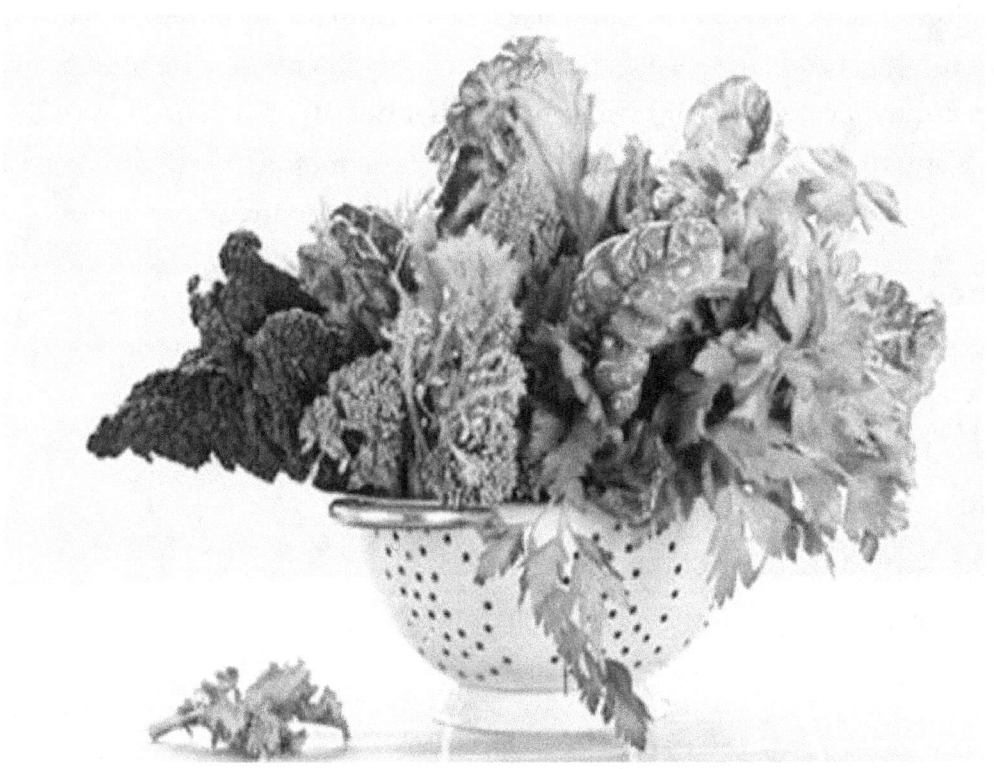

Follow Your Gut Feelings

Relieving Irritable Bowel Syndrome Naturally

Bishop Dr. Juliette D. Fagan

Copyright 2014 by All rights Reserved

Please Read:

This book and all of my other natural health related books are for educational purposes from a natural health perspective. *"Irritable Bowel Syndrome"* is based on natural health remedies using natural food as our medicine. It is not intended to be used as a substitute for medical advice or treatment. Neither does the book maker nor the author shall have any responsibility for any adverse reaction or effects arising directly or indirectly as a result of the information provided in this or any of my books.

Other books:

The Health Benefits of Coconut Oil, Water and Jelly

Let Food Be Your Medicine.

Websites:

www.healthysolutionsbiz.com
www.visionmiraclecog.info

About the Author

Bishop Dr. Juliette D. Fagan, Prof. A native born Caymanian, married to Pastor Leeroy Fagan. She is the owner and CEO of Healthy Solutions Colon Therapy and Detoxification Centre located in Jamaica and Grand Cayman. Dr. Fagan as she is affectionately called is a trained Practical Nurse, Cayman Islands School of Nursing, and Ex-Police Officer with The Royal Cayman Islands Police Force. She is also a gospel recording artist with two albums.

She studied Surgical Technology at Lindsey Hopkins Technical Miami Fla, Naturopathic Practitioner and Consultant at the Alternative Medicine of College of Canada, Colon Hydrotherapy, The International School for Colon Therapy USA, Clinical Colon Hydrotherapy, GI Doctors, Garden City NY with Amy Sanders of GPACT, she is Caribbean Ambassador of Global Professional Association for Colon Therapists.

She is a certified Prepare & Enrichment Family and Marital Counsellor Fla, Marriage officer Cayman Islands Government Bishop Dr. Fagan is the founder and President of Vision Miracle Churches of God Evangelistic Association and Vision Dominion School of Theology. A Graduate of the International Seminary USA, Professor of Theology, Christ Kingdom University Cameroon Africa. Radio and TV personality, author, inspirational, columnist and healthy life styles Speaker.

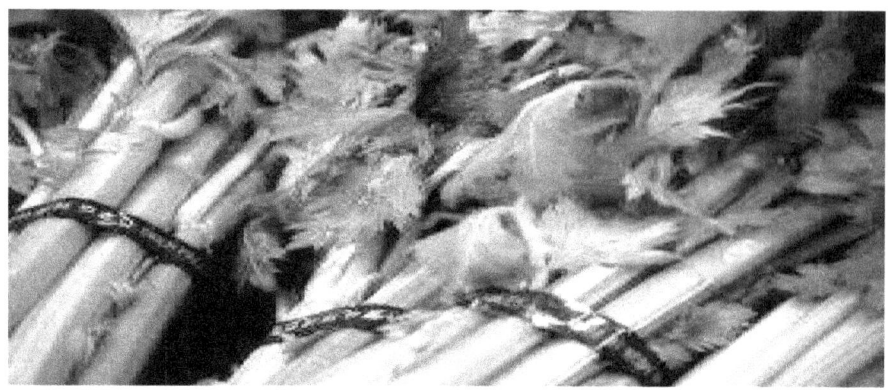

Acknowledgements:

It is an ongoing natural health crusade to educate, empower and bring hope to the minds and lives of thousands of people that really inspires me in one way or another. After publishing my first two books I realized that God didn't only call me to preach the gospel, but to also minister to the whole man using all of the knowledge and gifts He has blessed me with over the years as a nurse.

Thanks to the thousands of persons who will allow me to educate them to the truth not only spiritually, but also physically. To the Almighty God, I give thanks and praises for such blessings. Beth I did for you and so many others after listening to your plights with stomach and IBS issues. To all of my precious clients, thank you for your input. Thanks for your comments and reviews on facebook and tweeter, it has pushed me further. Pastor Ellen Peguero, Minister Elsa Bobb, Minister Jilliane Yunker, Dr Lloyd

Goldson, OB/GYN thanks for your encouragement over the years, your input continues to be very valuable to me…Sis Cynthia D. Johnson we did it (smile) your editing skills and assistance paid off indeed…thank you!

Leeroy you are my greatest inspiration babes, thanks for encouraging me to write more books, and for always giving such great testimonials at church, seminars and otherwise about how my books have helped you personally. Apart from God's blessings, you are one of the main reasons for my continued success in ministry and business wise. I don't have enough words to say how much I appreciate you.

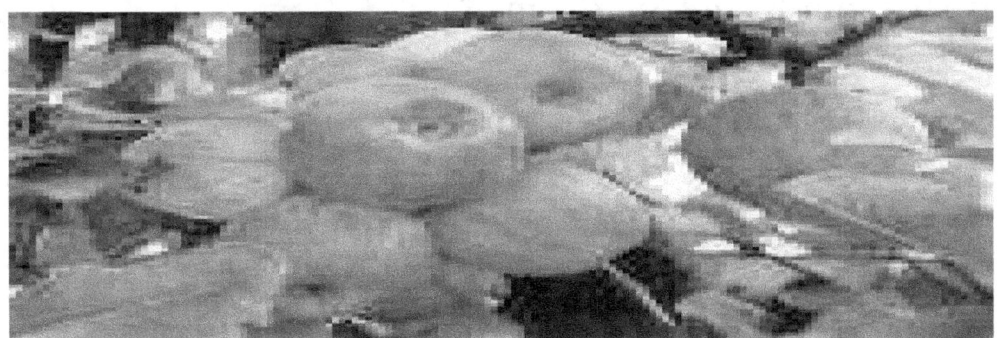

Table of Contents

Chapters

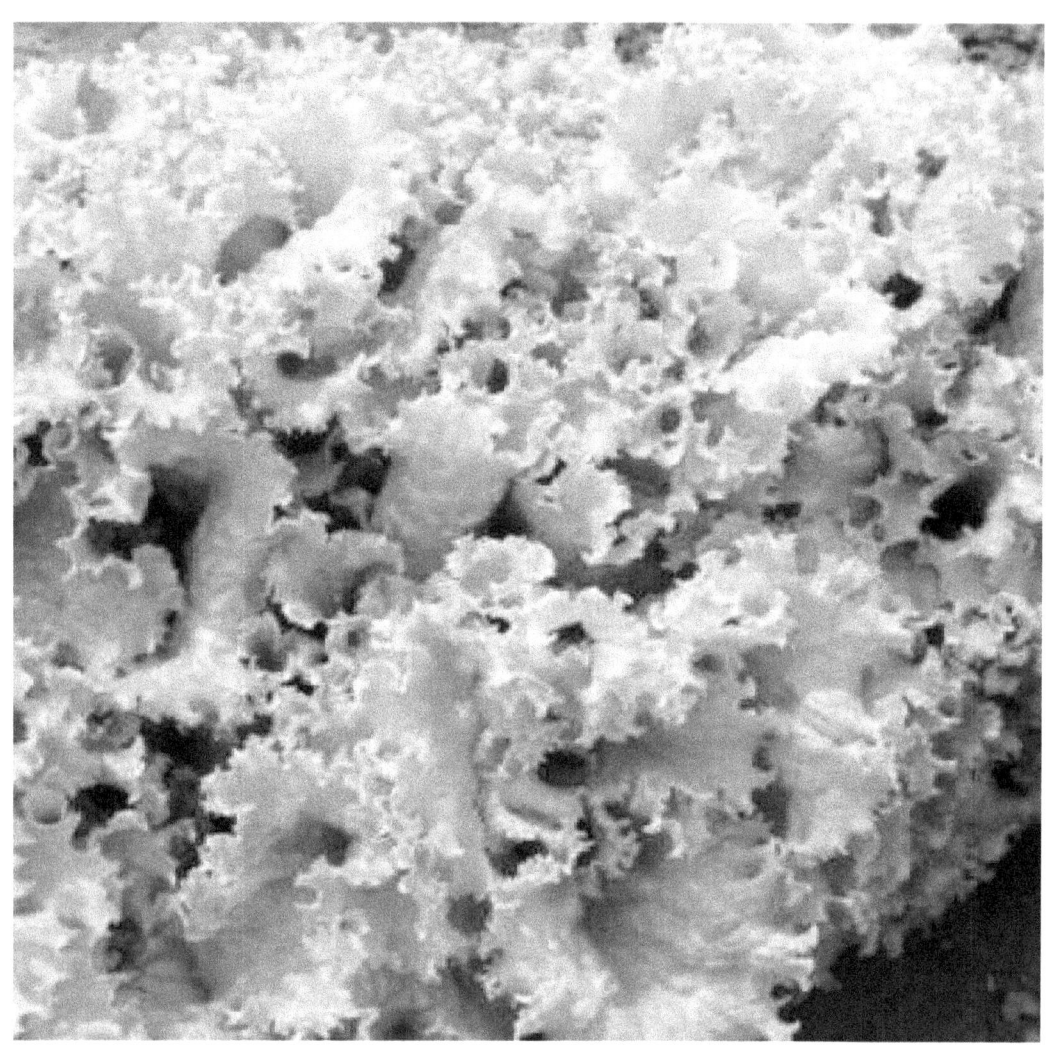

Natural Remedies To Optimum Health

Introduction

Everyone has an upset stomach from time to time. You probably know of the experience or someone with IBS – sometimes you've got gas and other times you feel nauseous or sick in your stomach. There may be times when you can't seem to go to the toilet for days due to constipations, then there are other days when diarrhea strikes and you can't stop going!

Although we all know that there are some foods or drinks that might trigger our digestive system to react in a certain way – a big meal of very spicy food sends many people rushing to the bathroom – the only really predictable thing about our digestive system is its unpredictability. However, because for most of us our digestive system acts the way we expect it to most of the time, we don't really give a great deal of thought to what our colon and gastrointestinal system is doing unless it is 'acting up'. I must say that this is not the case for everyone with IBS however.

As with the majority of non-life threatening medical conditions, there are essentially two ways that you can deal with IBS. First, option for most persons is to visit a medical doctor or other medical care professional, get a prescribed pharmaceutical medicine and take it. This option might be an effective way of easing your condition but as with many pharmaceutical situations and the drugs related to them, you have to consider the side effects also. The second alternative is to do things the natural way, dealing with your condition using only treatment methods and substances that in many examples have been used for hundreds and thousands of years. Let me make it clear, I am a naturopathic practitioner with several years of med-surgical nursing experience, so while I will highlight some medicines that your doctor is likely to prescribe for IBS and some possible side effects, the main focus of this book is not to tell you not to go to a medical doctor, but is giving you information for dealing with IBS naturally. In doing this, the idea is to encourage you to at least try to handle irritable bowel syndrome naturally before turning to chemical-based pharmaceutical drugs because dealing with the problem naturally is simply a better way to go.

What is Irritable Bowel Syndrome?

Irritable bowel syndrome is a chronic disorder (a long-term problem that could potentially last for life) IBS is a physical and not a psychological disorder that affects your gastrointestinal tract and intestines. It is a condition that is characterized by recurring problem in your stomach and bowels, often marked by regular bouts of diarrhea and / or constipation, stomach pain, spasms (cramps), bloating and gas etc. In effect, people who suffer from IBS have intestines that either squeeze too hard or do not squeeze hard enough to eject waste materials from their body. Thus, there is a lack of the normal continual rhythm that characterizes the average human digestive system. Research suggests that IBS sufferers appear to have a colon that is somehow more sensitive to a variety of different stimuli that have little or no effect on people who do not suffer from the condition. For example, certain foods that have no effect on other people can cause big problems for IBS sufferers. Furthermore, stress is also known to be an extremely important contributory factor for many sufferers. There is also some evidence that the immune system, the system in body that fights infection and disease is also somehow involved in the development of IBS.

Irritable bowel syndrome is a condition that most commonly hits people between the years of 20 and 30.

One of the major difficulties attached to dealing with the problem is that while many of the symptoms are easily recognizable, the actual cause of irritable bowels syndrome has not been fully understood. For example, there are no specific signs of physical disease in the colon of most IBS sufferers, and there are no specific tests that can be used to diagnose the condition either. Nevertheless, it is a fact that for many IBS sufferers, the symptoms do deteriorate after eating or when they are under stress, so this is a consideration which most doctors takes into account when attempting to diagnose whether you are suffering from irritable bowel syndrome or not.

In addition, irritable bowel syndrome is not really one recognizable medical condition at all as the term is used as a blanket to cover many different medicals symptoms that would usually be seen as nothing more than an upset stomach was they to occur in isolation.

What this means is that every imaginable symptom that you could possibly conceive of as a result of suffering an upset stomach is a symptom that you can associate with irritable bowel syndrome. As suggested, IBS is a condition that can persist for many years, but the good news is, the disorder itself does not tend to get more serious or severe overtime.

It is said that individual IBS 'attacks' can vary in severity, the condition itself does not. Furthermore, under normal circumstances, IBS has nothing to do with and does not lead to more serious medical conditions such as cancer or inflammatory bowel disease. As a natural health educator, let me inform you that if you ever see a reference to mucus colitis, nervous diarrhea, spastic colon or spastic colitis, you can be sure that it is referring in some way to irritable bowel syndrome.

When to Eat If You Have IBS

If you actually knew just how many people were dealing with irritable bowels syndrome at any given time, you would probably be shocked. As a matter of fact, it is considered that up to 50% of all individuals are suffering or will suffer from some kind of IBS symptoms at some point in their life but many of them will never seek medical attention. The simple fact of the matter is, there is not a single problem that is identified as being irritable bowel syndrome, and it could be a number of different problems that you may be dealing with.

If you are having or have had irritable bowel syndrome for quite some time, you probably already recognize the fact that the foods that you eat are going to affect your symptoms in some way or another. More often than not, you will recognize whenever foods are a problem, as your symptoms to become worse but you might be surprised to learn that you may also be eating foods which are causing your irritable bowel syndrome symptoms to go away to a certain extent. Just because you don't recognize that is the fact, does not necessarily mean that it is not true.

Believe it or not, it also has a lot to do with when you eat as well as what you eat in order to affect your irritable bowel syndrome to your benefit. For example, most of us tend to eat meals whenever we have the opportunity and it is very rare that we actually sit down to eat a meal at the same time each day. If you are dealing with symptoms of irritable bowel syndrome, however, it is important for you to make sure that you are eating regularly, whenever that happens to be for you.

It is also important for you to split up your meals into smaller batches if you are having a difficult time with diarrhea. Many times, just eating smaller meals throughout the day may be enough to help you to overcome a problem with diarrhea. The opposite, however, is also true and if you are suffering from constipation as a result of your irritable bowel syndrome then you might want to eat three larger meals every day and include plenty of natural fiber in those meals. This along with plenty water is good for constipation and to get things moving along properly again.

Balancing Your Enzymes for IBS Relief

The body is truly an amazing machine that was uniquely created by God, and whenever it is working properly, we rarely ever have to worry about any problems that may be occurring on the outside because of issues on the inside. The unfortunate thing is, we live in a world that does not necessarily promote a healthy lifestyle or give us what we need in order to be as balanced as possible. Trying to live and eat healthy can be a challenge for many because of the high cost for organic foods.

We tend to be bombarded by things that are bad for us, both in the environment around us and also in the foods that we eat and the water that we most times have to drink. For quite a few individuals, this results in irregularity and other irritable bowel syndrome symptoms.

Believe it or not, it is not all that difficult for you to use food as your medicine to cure your irritable bowel syndrome and to remove many of the symptoms that you may be experiencing. It really has to do with the balance that is on the inside of your body, however delicate that balance may be.

The unfortunate thing about IBS is, until now medical science is really unable to determine why persons develop or have IBS in the first place. From what I have heard, they simply tend to lump all of the different symptoms into the same category, even though they are obviously different problems. For example, I have heard clients say they were told their problem with diarrhea is irritable bowel syndrome while also calling constipation the same thing.

If you really want to get rid of your irritable bowel syndrome symptoms, you need to make sure that the natural balance within your body is as perfect as possible. First of all, I need to let you know that it is going to be impossible for you to balance this perfectly. Because of various farming techniques and the imperfection of man, it is impossible for you to get these enzymes as they were actually meant to exist in the body. Even so, you can typically give your body what it needs if you feed it properly.

This can be a little bit difficult for a person with IBS, especially considering that many of these enzymes will come to you in raw fruits and vegetables. That is why it may be necessary for you to supplement regularly in order to bring this balance back to your body (gut) until you can begin to take them in naturally. This can be done through natural yogurts, vitamins and probiotics that are available through a health food store. It may take a little bit of experimentation to find something that won't upset you but once you find it, you will feel the road to recovery.

Food Allergies - IBS Triggers

Do you have a difficulty with irritable bowel syndrome? If you do, remember you are not alone, as the vast majority of people are going to suffer from these difficulties at some point in their life or another. From what I understand, pinpointing exactly what is causing the IBS problems can be a little bit difficult. One of the main reasons why this is the case is because so many different problems can be lumped together under the same disease. For example, a problem with diarrhea is considered to be dealing with the same thing as a person with constipation. Understanding this makes it obvious why treating or dealing with the problem of irritable bowel syndrome is so difficult.

Believe it or not, you may have a difficulty with irritable bowel syndrome but the reason that you are actually suffering is because of the trigger that is causing the symptoms to come to the front. If you are able to keep these symptoms under control, the disease would still be going on in the background but you would not have to deal with it because of not triggering the events from taking place which caused the difficulty. Thus far it seems, that one of the main things that triggers IBS problems are food allergies.

There are a number of different food allergies that could lead to problems with irritable bowel syndrome. For example, many people are allergic to nuts and while some of them may be allergic to the point where it ends up with a death causing situation, other people may be mildly allergic so that they are only having IBS symptoms after eating the nuts. Milk is also another problem that causes these conditions regularly and many people are lactose intolerant, unable to digest the proteins that are contained in cow's milk.

If you regularly have a problem with the irritable bowel syndrome, one of the best things that you can do is to keep track of all of the foods that you are eating, along with any symptoms that you may be experiencing. By doing this, you will be able to determine which foods are causing the problems in you and then avoid them so you do not have those problems flaring up regularly. It may sound simplistic, but it's one of the best ways for you to be able to overcome a problem with irritable bowel symptoms once and for all.

Eating at Regular Times

The human body is not only amazing in the way that it is uniquely designed and the things it does, it is also rather interesting. There are times whenever things that may go wrong with the body, such as irritable bowel syndrome, which may be able to be overcome. There are some things that can be done naturally, however, which have been shown to help in these cases. For example eating at regular times and eating the right food may help you to deal with the issue successfully.

Although this seems like it would be an easy thing to put into practice, the majority of us do not have an easy time eating at regular times. The reason why this is often the case is because all of us tend to be busy people and there are plenty of times whenever it is more convenient for us to put off a meal than to eat right, drink water or even use the toilet. For those who suffer from irritable bowel syndrome symptoms, however, it may be a small thing to do in order to overcome the flare up.

Something else that you may need to do is to change the amount of times that you eat every day in order to help you overcome the symptoms. Since irritable bowel can cause a number of different problems in us that range all the way from diarrhea to constipation, varying the times that we eat from five times a day all the way down to two or three, may have an effect on it.

Most people find that if they have diarrhea, this is easily overcome by eating several small meals throughout the day instead of eating the typical two or three meals per day. The opposite is also true of those who suffer from constipation and eating a couple of larger meals every day which includes plenty of fiber may be able to help you in this instance. It may seem unusual that this is the case but you would be surprised with how effective it can be to change the times that you are eating throughout the day or simply to just eat at the same time every day on a regular basis. Once the body gets used to something like this, it affects everything about us which would include our digestive process. It's a small price to pay to overcome something as uncomfortable as IBS.

Do You Need More Stomach Acid?

You would probably be surprised at the number of individuals that suffer in this way on a regularly basis. At times, the solution to this problem may be as simple as having more digestive juices available for you in order to help the process along. Since digestion is in its early phases whatever it is in the stomach, it is reasonable to conclude that having more stomach acid may be able to help us to digest our food more easily that it can be absorbed by the body.

This can also be seen in another way. Believe it or not, heartburn is caused by a lack of stomach acid of the system and although many people would think that this was the opposite, that isn't the case at all. That is why most of the medications that you take for heartburn need to be taken for your entire life, because they don't really solve the problem of low stomach acid, they just really treat the symptom of heartburn you have because of it. And by taking anti-acids it only makes matters worst.

If you want to be able to overcome your irritable bowel syndrome symptoms, which could also include heartburn, one thing that you want to do is to build up the amount of stomach acid that you have in your system naturally. Believe it or not, this is not all that difficult to do; many people find it to be a pleasure once they understand the way to cure the problem.

Getting more greens in your system is one way for you to be able to build up your stomach acid to normal levels. This can be difficult, and it can actually be uncomfortable for somebody that is suffering from irritable bowel syndrome. That is, of course, unless they get those greens in the form of a green smoothie. Here's how you make one.

You start with two pieces of your favorite fruit, it really doesn't matter which two pieces you use. You would then mix those two pieces with a large handful of green, leafy vegetables and some water with ice in it. Blend it all until it is smooth a then add a little bit of honey if additional sweetness is desired. Drink one of these every day, and your body will get the greens that it needs in order to build up your stomach acid and get rid of your symptoms. You can also get more ideas on the health benefits fresh raw juices from my book "Let Food Be Your Medicine" and "The natural health benefits of coconut oil, water and jelly" I also heard from few persons that fennel tea, peppermint oil also soothes and relaxes the tummy.

Lactose Intolerance and IBS

There are a number of different conditions that can occur within the human body that, although they are not deadly or dangerous, they can be quite uncomfortable. A good example of this is if you suffer from irritable bowel syndrome but you might be interested in knowing that even though it may hurt to suffer from this, it is not something that is going to cause any permanent damage in most cases. As I said before, medical science is really unable to tell exactly what causes your irritable bowel syndrome, but they do recognize the fact that there may be triggers which can cause it to flare or get worse.

Whenever you go in to have a test done in order to see if you have irritable bowels syndrome, it is going to be determined by a process of elimination, rather than being a part of a test that will actually help you to determine if you have the problem. As a matter of fact, many of the problems that can be experienced by IBS sufferers may also be the exact same problems that could be caused by a number of other health issues, some of them which are rather serious.

One of the things that may mimic irritable bowel syndrome in us is intolerance to drinking cow's milk. This is actually a fairly common problem and many of us are unable to digest the proteins that are in the cow's milk and we have a condition that is known as lactose intolerance. It could be that you are not suffering from irritable bowel syndrome at all but, in reality, you are suffering from an inability to digest milk and milk products. If that is the case, the cure for your irritable bowel syndrome symptoms might mean you just need to avoid milk.

There may also be times, however, when you are suffering from lactose intolerance along with a problem with irritable bowel syndrome. If this is the case with you, the lactose intolerance will act as a trigger that can cause the irritable bowel syndrome symptoms to get much worse. In order for you to overcome it, you can either reduce the amount of milk that you are drinking or get rid of it altogether, and you should see some significant relief.

Avoiding Problem Foods

Whenever most people begin having problems with irritable bowel syndrome, it tends to catch them somewhat by surprise. It certainly has an uncomfortable feel to it and in many cases; it can be quite severe, at times to the point where you may think that you have other more complicated problems. That is why it is important for you to be tested in order to make sure that the irritable bowel syndrome symptoms that you have are not part of a more serious problem, such as Cohn's disease or ulcerative colitis (some kind of inflammation or bleeding in the colon).

Once it has been determined that you are dealing with irritable bowel syndrome, there are a number of different things that you may be able to do which will reduce the amount of suffering and discomfort that you are feeling regularly. Believe it or not, one of the main things that can be done is to avoid things that are causing the problems to trigger in the first place. Although you may not be able to get rid of IBS altogether, by reducing the triggers down to a minimum, you can reduce the suffering down to a minimum right along with it.

Many of the triggers that are experienced by those who suffer from IBS include the foods that they eat. This can either be because of a food allergy or because of an inability of the human body to be able to successfully digest these foods.

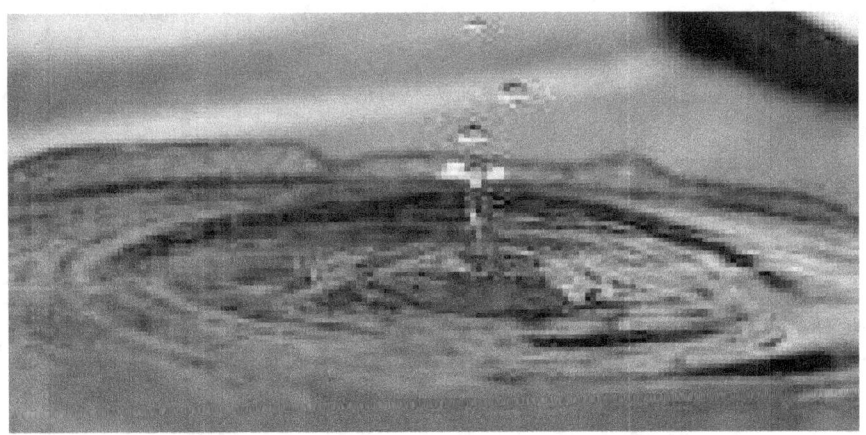

Why Water Can Relieve IBS

There are many different functions that go on within the human body that are completely under the radar. A good example of this is the digestive process and many of us really don't give any thought to the fact that the food that we eat is broken down on the chemical level so that we are able to be energized from the nutrients that it contains. Whenever this digestive process is working properly, it does not typically give us any problems but whenever something goes wrong, those problems can be rather uncomfortable. If you have IBS think about your colon also.

A classic example of this is the way that the food is passed through the large intestines and eventually expelled from the body. The large intestine will contract rhythmically in order to push the food through and to expel some additional nutrients from it along the way. Whenever we are suffering from irritable bowel syndrome, these contractions become erratic and may actually become uncomfortable. There may be times whenever the food is rapidly pushed through and expelled, a condition that is known as rapid transit. Whenever the food travels through are colon quickly, we can also experience diarrhea. When it passes through too slowly, constipation is typically a problem.

You might not believe this, but a simple way for you to be able to correct many of the problems that are associated with irritable bowel syndrome is to drink plenty of water. One of the reasons why these contractions are occurring irregularly may be as a result of the body trying to get additional water out of the feces because you're not giving enough in a natural way. The colon or large intestine absorbs water every couple minute. Lack of water is one of the main causes of constipation and simply drinking enough water on a daily basis can help to prevent constipation.

Once most of us understand that the water that is fueling our body is coming from the feces it becomes a little bit easier for us to drink more water in order to overcome the problem. What you need to do, however, is to drink half of your body weight every day in ounces of water in order to be properly hydrated. Unless you have high blood pressure, you should also take some sea salt without water in order to allow it to stay in your body long enough to do its work. Most people receive relief from their IBS after just a few days of doing this water treatment. Continue to do it for the rest of your life, and you may be able to live a life free of your symptoms altogether.

Natural remedies for IBS

Irritable bowel syndrome is a very uncomfortable problem that far too many people experience on a regular basis. Unfortunately, most people tend to live with this condition for the majority of their lives, not really knowing what it is that can be done in order to overcome it. The simple fact of the matter is, IBS is not a disease that is life threatening, but it is certainly something that is curable if you understand a few basics about the human body.

Here are 3 different things that can with your IBS. The first thing that may be able to relieve your IBS is getting enough water to drink. Most of us tend to be dehydrated and some of us may have been chronically dehydrated for the majority of our lives.

The body is going to attempt to get water from any source that it possibly can in order to fuel itself if you're not giving it to it in the proper way. As I said before, one way this is done is by squeezing water out of the feces as it travels through the colon. Hydrate yourself properly by drinking plenty of water on a daily basis and you will not only notice IBS relief, this unsavory condition will cease.

Something else that may be needed and can often help with your irritable bowel syndrome quickly is to build up the stomach acids that may be lacking. Not only can low stomach acid cause irritable bowel syndrome, it is also the primary cause of heartburn and acid reflux. The way that you build up stomach acid is fairly simple; you need to eat greener, leafy vegetables every day. The best way for you to do this is in the form of a green smoothie or juice which is a combination of two pieces of fruit, a large handful of greens that is all blended with water and a bit of ice. Drink these daily and get relief.

Finally, you might want to consider giving up milk and milk products altogether for a while to see what happens. No matter what the mainstream media wants to teach to you, cow's milk is not something that is healthy for you as none of us are cows. Because of an inability of the human body to digest cow's milk properly, different symptoms may occur which can not only mimic irritable bowel syndrome, it can irritate the existing problem. Remove or reduce your milk consumption considerably and you will see a difference in the way that you feel quickly. Try almond or rice milk and see what happens.

Exercise and Irritable Bowel Syndrome

There are several different things that can be done which can improve the overall health of humans but unfortunately, very few of us take the time to make sure that we are doing them on a regular basis. One of these things is exercise and although the majority of us realize the fact that exercise is good for us, we may not take the time to do so because of a busy schedule or a lack of interest in pushing our body to the limit. You might be interested in knowing, however, that it not only can help you to feel better overall, it may help you to treat problems such as irritable bowel syndrome.

One of the things that exercise is to the body is an overall agent that will help to reduce any problems that you may be experiencing. It is a great stress reliever, which tends to be a major trigger for individuals that are suffering from irritable bowel syndrome. It also helps the entire digestive process and if you do a mild exercise soon after you eat by walking, you can actually help the digestive process and get things moving along to start out with. In itself, this is often enough to remove the irritable bowel syndrome symptoms that you may be experiencing.

It is not necessary for you to exercise extensively in order to see results from doing this. As a matter of fact, just getting anywhere from 20 to 30 minutes of brisk walking in on a daily basis is often enough to make a difference in how you feel and the symptoms that you experience. Best of all, this doesn't need to be done all at one time and you can often achieve the same results by exercising for five or 10 minute intervals all throughout the day.

If you have never exercise before, you have not experienced the life-changing effects that it can have on the human body. Of course, once you do begin to exercise you would want to make sure that you are staying hydrated as you will be losing excess water. This can also affect the amount of irritable bowel syndrome symptoms that you are experiencing. Make sure that you start and make it a part of your regular life; you will experience great relief from your symptoms and feel better overall.

Your IBS and Milk

There may be times when ever we are suffering from a problem in our body and it might be as a result of something that we are not even thinking about. For example, many of us suffer from irritable bowel syndrome regularly that can result in things such as diarrhea, constipation, gas and severe bloating. The discomfort that often goes along with IBS is quite severe and in some cases, can be debilitating to a certain extent. The fortunate thing is, irritable bowel syndrome is not a deadly problem but whenever you're suffering from it, it bears looking into.

The reason why this is a case is because many people that think they are suffering from irritable bowel syndrome may not actually have a problem with it at all. There are plenty of other things that can give the same symptoms that are experienced by someone with IBS, some of which are more severe and others which are simply a matter of being a food allergy.

A perfect example of this is somebody that is lactose intolerant. These people may suffer from many of the same symptoms that are associated with irritable bowel syndrome. Most people that cut milk out of their diet may miss it for a little while but eventually, the cravings will disappear and best of all, the irritable bowel syndrome symptoms that they are experiencing will disappear right along with them.

Things That Cause IBS

If you are suffering from irritable bowel syndrome, one of the only ways for you to end your suffering is to remove the things that are triggering the symptoms in the first place. The unfortunate thing is, these triggers may be quite varied and depending on you as an individual, it could be one thing when it could be something entirely different in somebody else. Even though this is the case, however, there are some common triggers that are easy to identify and when you identify them, its best you deal with them quickly.

Another thing that causes problems with IBS in many individuals is dehydration, particularly when you have a problem with constipation. Not everybody that suffers from irritable bowel syndrome is going to suffer from constipation and many of them may have diarrhea instead. Whenever your stool is hard and dry, however, it may be as a direct result of the body trying to squeeze water out of it in order to provide the body with fluids as a result of being dehydrated. This is a rather unsavory thought, and it is the cause of a lot of diseases that we may be suffering from. Make sure that you drink plenty of water and keep yourself hydrated regularly and you should see the symptoms disappearing. That's why I highly recommend persons with IBS to have colon therapy done followed by probiotics.

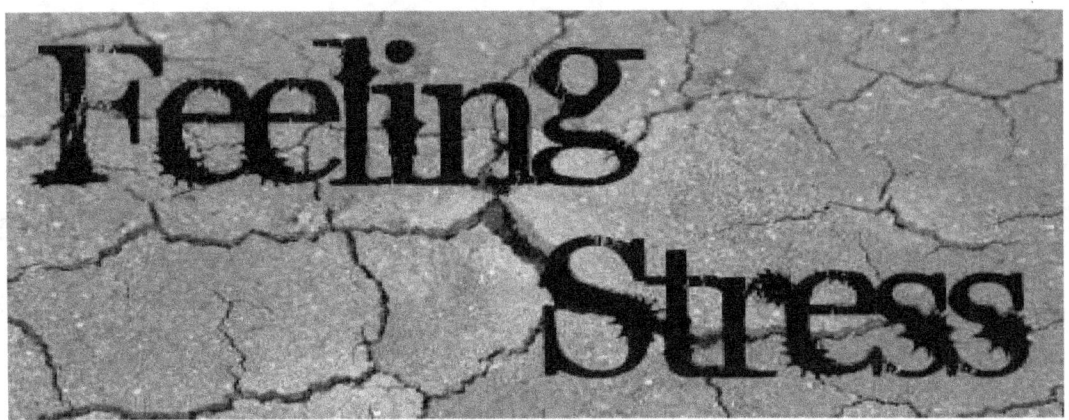

The Stress Factor

Another thing that this not necessarily the cause of irritable bowel syndrome but it certainly is a trigger is stress. People today are stressed regularly and it may be very difficult for you to avoid having the stress, simply because it is a part of our lives. In order to overcome these problems, it is necessary for you to find coping mechanisms that will keep the stress from welling up in you and causing your irritable bowel problems. This is just another way that you can reduce your discomfort and the symptoms that you are experiencing. Stress sends off its own chemicals and can trigger other ailments in the body.

The Connection of Probiotics and IBS

There are many different systems that are at work inside of the body at any given time and in order for the body to be functioning properly, all of these needs to be working properly. A good example of this is the digestive system and for any number of different reasons, this system may become disrupted and problems, such as irritable bowel syndrome can occur. A prime example of why you may be experiencing some of these problems is because of a lack of flora and fauna that is in the digestive tract. Without this, it will be impossible for you to digest your food properly. I have a wonderful teaching in my book "Let Food Be Your Medicine" I suggest you get it also.

These living products (gut flora), along with a variety of different enzymes that should be in proportion within us at any given time help to keep this delicate system in balance within our body. Irritable bowel syndrome, unfortunately, is experienced by far too many individuals that do not have this balance in place. In order for you to overcome the symptoms that you may be experiencing, it is often necessary for you to bring your system back into a balance that it may have lost over the course of time. This can either be as a result of dietary problems, dehydration, medication, constipation or perhaps the prolonged use of antibiotics.

Believe it or not, bringing this balance back and overcoming many of your irritable bowel syndrome symptoms can be as simple as taking a very tiny pill every day. This pill comes in the form of what is commonly known as a probiotic and it gives your digestive system many of the enzymes that it needs in order to grow and Flora and fauna. In doing so, it helps your body to be able to digest the food properly and to extract the nutrients from the things that you eat in order to keep your body healthy. It also has the effect, in many cases, of reducing the painful symptoms that are associated with IBS.

It is important to note that not all probiotics are going to be created equally and some of them may be a little bit more commercial than others. Since you are dealing with something that is all-natural (organic), make sure that is created by a company that puts a lot of emphasis on the natural goodness of their products. In doing so, you will have the best opportunity of overcoming the problems that you are experiencing and restoring your overall digestive health.

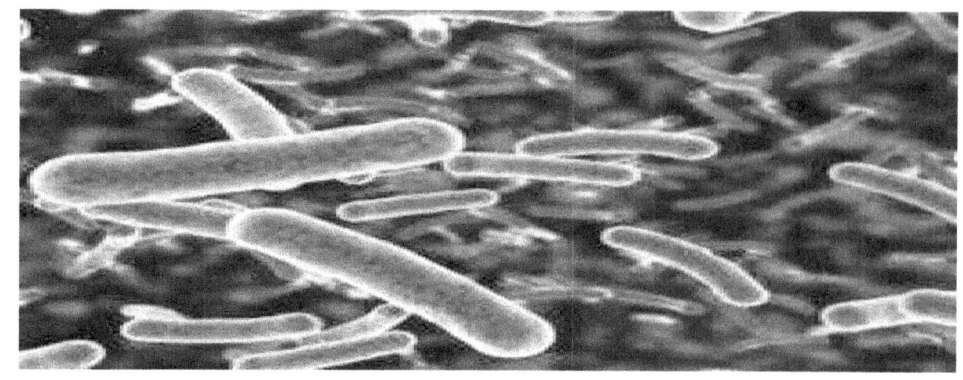

Treating Irritable Bowel Syndrome Naturally

Whenever the human body is really working well, we rarely ever experience difficulties that are associated with irritable bowel syndrome. The unfortunate fact of the matter is whenever we have digestive problems, sometimes the stomach problem is lumped together into one category and refer to as being IBS. In reality, however, there are a number of different conditions that can cause this difficulty, and the symptoms that go along with it which can range from bloating to diarrhea or perhaps even the opposite, constipation.

In order to overcome the difficulties with your irritable bowel syndrome one of two things is generally needed. We either need to remove something from our day to day activities that is triggering the symptoms that we are experiencing or we need to add something to our body that it may be lacking in order to help us to effectively overcome these conditions.

Many of the things that we need to remove from our system in order to overcome irritable bowel syndrome come in the form of food. Food allergies are very common but unfortunately, most people don't recognize the fact that they have these allergies in the first place. Have you ever noticed that you are congested after you eat, perhaps with a runny nose or a feeling as if you need to clear your throat? These are classic food allergies but in more severe forms, they can easily cause problems with irritable bowel syndrome. Keep a record of what you eat and how it reacts with your body if you are experiencing certain stomach problems. Very quickly, you will be able to determine things that need to be removed from your diet. As far as adding things to your body in order to keep it running properly, there are a few things that can be done to correct irritable bowel syndrome.

Dehydration is one of the main problems which cause this condition so staying hydrated properly may be able to help you overcome it quickly.

Low stomach acid is also something which may cause this condition so getting plenty of greens into your diet can help you to build back up normal stomach acid levels again.

Finally, you will want to improve your overall digestive health by taking a natural probiotic once or twice every day. This will not only help you to build up your enzyme levels but it will help you to restore your natural Flora and fauna which will keep away the symptoms that you are experiencing.

Dealing with Depression

There are many of who have to deal with irritable bowel syndrome symptoms from time to time but it could not be anything that would really be considered chronic. Occasional bouts with diarrhea, constipation, upset stomach, gas or bloating might simply be shrugged off as eating the wrong thing or perhaps those we are sick. Some of us, however, have IBS to the point where it is chronic and debilitating. This can not only change our lifestyle considerably, it can also be quite depressing because of the lifestyle changes that we are experiencing. If you are depressed over irritable bowel syndrome, what can be done to overcome this depression? Bear in mind that there are many things that can cause depression.

There are several different ways of coping with depression, especially when you have problems with your digestive health. You might be surprised to learn that many of the ways of helping you to overcome this depression may actually also assist you in overcoming your digestive problems as well. Here are a couple of different ways that you may be able to treat your depression effectively and if you work at these regularly, you may be able to improve your digestive health and remove the source of the depression at the same time.

One of the most important things for somebody that is depressed to do is to eat right and exercise regularly. The unfortunate thing is this can also be one of the more difficult things for them to do because of the way that they are feeling. Exercise is fantastic for helping you with depression and not only does it do so by strengthening your overall body and mental capacities, it also releases chemicals into your body that act as endorphins. These make you feel good while you're exercising and can help you to feel good even after you stop.

Something else that is important for you to do is to make sure that you are treating your overall health with love and respect. Getting plenty of rest at night, drinking enough water to stay hydrated and eating the proper foods can not only help with your depressed mental attitude, it can also help with your digestive health. Prayer, praise and worship, thankfulness and having faith in God has also been proven to help some people. The mere fact that some people are alive causes them to be thankful. It might be odd to some, but that these things would go hand-in-hand but that's the beauty of it as well. By working on things that will improve our depressed mental outlook on life, in many cases we are able to remove our digestive and other health problems which can be the source of that depression in the first place.

Natural coconut oil is also an excellent source of oil that can also help with your digestive health and assist you in overcoming any irritable bowel syndrome symptoms that you may be experiencing. Make sure that you include coconut oil, coconut water and coconut milk in your daily routine and you will find that those symptoms are disappearing. Stay away from egg, soy diary, gluten and yeast products. Trans (bad) fat is found in all processed and boxed food.

Massage Therapy and IBS

There are a number of different healthy things that can be done which can not only improve our overall general health; they may be able to help us with some very specific problems that we are experiencing. For example, if you are having a trouble with irritable bowel syndrome, which is very common, you might be surprised with exactly how effective massages can be in helping you to overcome it. What type of massages should you be getting and how can these assist you in overcoming your problem?

The digestive system is truly amazing and it is not always as a result of our colon having problems that these digestive issues are occurring. In many cases, it can be as a result of low stomach acid or perhaps other issues, such as food allergies or perhaps dehydration. Regardless of why you are having these issues, massage can assist you to overcome them and in some remarkable ways. For example, massage can help to relieve the body and to bring a flow of energy back to it that may be lacking. Getting regular massages can promote healthy energy flow in the body.

Another issue that may help you as far as a massage is concerned is the relaxation benefits that are typically experienced. Massages are not all about the body and as a matter of fact, the mind is affected even more than the body in many cases. By helping us to relieve the stress that we may be experiencing, we can remove one of the largest triggers of irritable bowel syndrome that we may be experiencing. Most people find this to be a pleasurable experience and it helps them to be able to cope with life, along with coping with digestive problems. Regardless of why it is that massage can help you to overcome your irritable bowel syndrome, the fact is that it seems to be able to help in almost every case. Why not try getting regular massages for yourself? You will enjoy the benefits that come your way.

The Master Cleanse

As stated before, there are many different ways for you to overcome IBS naturally but in some cases, it may take a little bit more effort than others. For example, if you are dealing with chronic irritable bowel syndrome, it might be necessary for you to cleanse your entire body in order to remove those problems.

Apart from the hydro therapy or colon therapy, one of the best cleanses that can be done for irritable bowel syndrome or any other health condition that you may be dealing with in general is the master cleanse. This is not the easiest thing that you're ever going to do but if you can successfully stay on it for duration, you will notice major differences in your health. Throughout the day, you can have anywhere from 10 to 12 glasses of the following:

Mix 8 to 10 ounces of water with two tablespoons of organic fresh squeezed lemon juice, organic / raw maple syrup or molasses and a healthy pinch of cayenne pepper. This will be your only food or drink that you can have through the day, other than pure or coconut water.

In the morning, you will have a saltwater flush of 1 quart of pure water with two tablespoons of sea salt (**WARNING:** If you have high blood pressure no kind of salt drink).
Before you go to bed, drink a cup of herbal laxative tea. These two

things help to keep the system moving, even with the lack of fiber in your diet.

The reason why the master cleanse is so effective at helping you to clean your colon and to maintain your colon health is because it reset your entire system. The cravings that you have for things that are bad for you will disappear during the master cleanse and you will receive a mental and physical clarity that you have never experienced before. It's an experience that I highly recommend and if you have a problem with IBS, it can be an experience that is life changing. I have done the master cleanse for years with great results.

The Benefits of Green Smoothies

There are so many different things that can go wrong with the human body and our digestive health. That is why many individuals experience irritable bowel syndrome at some point in their life, along with other symptoms that may be related, such as heartburn and acid reflux. In order to overcome these problems, it is necessary for you to promote digestive health of the body that may be much stricter than what you are used to. In reality, however, it only has to do in many cases with the level of stomach acid and the amount of gut flora.

Let me make it clear, I'm not talking about a regular fruit smoothie, but I'm talking about what is referred to as a green smoothie, a smoothie with maybe one apple and a large handful of leafy, green vegetables added. This is a delicious drink and when made properly, it is tastier than a regular fruit smoothie. Best yet, it has all of the healthy greens that you need in order to get through the day in a form that your body can easily assimilate.

After just a few days of enjoying these green smoothies, the stomach acid will begin to regulate itself and many of the problems that you have with your digestion will begin to correct themselves naturally. One of the more interesting, and unusable things about irritable bowel syndrome is the fact that there are so many different symptoms that may be associated with it.

For example, some people may experience diarrhea whenever they have IBS and others may be the exact opposite and experience constipation. Obviously, these do not stem from the same exact causes so it may be necessary for you to treat your irritable bowel syndrome according to the symptoms that you have. Eat smaller meals for IBS diarrhea and more fiber for constipation.

Before You Do Colon Therapy

One of the things that are commonly used in order to restore our digestive health is to have a colonic done. A well trained therapist will inform you of the cons and pros of colon hydrotherapy. A colonic, colon irrigation or colon therapy is basically a higher form of enema, a procedure in which the entire colon (descending, transverse and ascending colon) is soaked with warm filtered water through a small speculum inserted in the rectum to remove impacted feces. This is a natural health procedure that can have a profound effect on our overall health. Feces left in the colon for too long can lead to various diseases including irritable bowel syndrome and leaky gut. I will explain more in another book as it pertains to colon therapy.

I think I said it before but will say it again, it is your responsibility to make sure that you trust the person that is giving you the colonic (or treating you for that matter), as there are some people who are administering colon therapy (and other treatments) who can actually cause more harm than good. As a Global Professional Association for Colon Therapy (GPACT) Certified and Clinically Trained Colon Therapist, one of the reasons I was approved by the governing bodies is because I am aware of the benefits and also the various contraindications of colon therapy.

Colon therapy is not for everyone. You also want to make sure the therapist has knowledge about aseptic techniques, sterility and are using FDA approved disposable speculums and tubing, and that the water they are using is warm, pure, filtered and the equipment is FDA approved for colonics. A regular colonic, when administered properly can restore the natural rhythmic contraction of the colon and remove many of the problems that we are having with IBS.

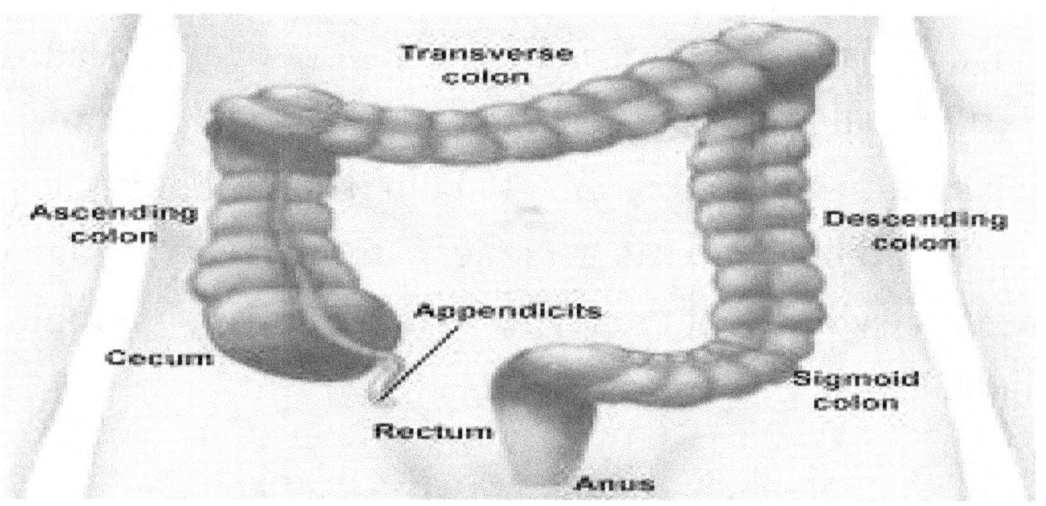

Conclusion:

Of course, these are only some of the things that may be done which can help to improve your IBS symptoms. You also want to make sure that you're eating the right kind of foods, drinking plenty of water, boosting your immune system, rest, exercise and doing things regularly that will also improve your digestive health.

If you can just learn to care your gut, you will see a difference in how many episodes of IBS you have and your overall health in general. So glad I was able to share with you and I pray and trust you have learnt a few more things about irritable bowel syndrome and how you can get relief naturally. I encourage you to spread the word about relieving irritable bowel syndrome naturally.

Ask…Believe…Receive!

Exodus 23:25
Worship the LORD your God, and his blessing will be on your food and water. I will take away sickness from among you,

Psalm 30:2
O LORD my God, I called to you for help and you healed me.

Isaiah 53:4-5

surely, he took up our infirmities and carried our sorrows, yet we considered him stricken by God, smitten by him, and afflicted. But he was pierced for our transgressions, he was crushed for our iniquities; the punishment that brought us peace was upon him, and by his wounds we are healed.

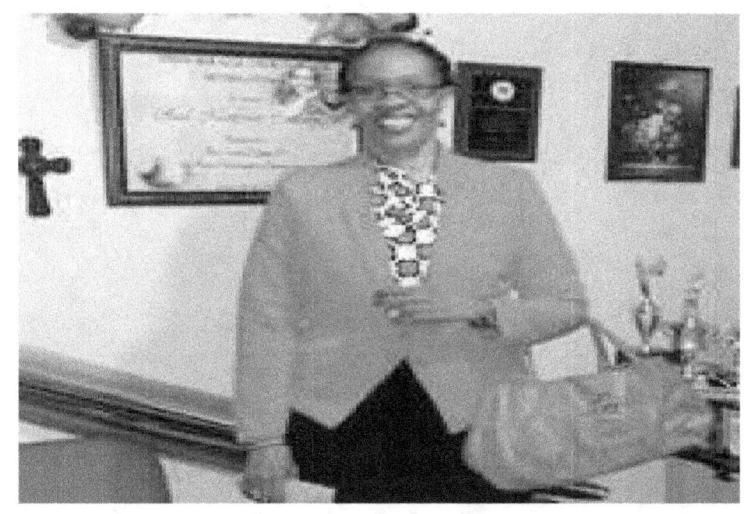

Thank You for Purchasing My Books!

Bishop Dr Juliette Dr. Fagan

www.healthysolutionsbiz.com

www.visionmiraclecog.info

Tel: 1876 469-3973, 1876 783-2378, 1876 456-8444

Copyright 2014

www.ingramcontent.com/pod-product-compliance
Lightning Source LLC
Chambersburg PA
CBHW080444290526
45791CB00008BA/2607